Cascade of Tears

The Journey through Chronic Illness and Pain

LACRESHA N. HAYES

ISBN: 978-0-9886772-6-5

Unless otherwise noted, all Scripture quotations are
from the King James Version of the Bible.

Publisher is Lanico Media House, imprint of Lanico
Enterprise.

Printed in the United States of America.

DEDICATION AND ACKNOWLEDGMENT

For all those who have struggled to regain control after being rocked by chronic illness. You are not alone.

Special thank you to my former primary care physician, Dr. David Foscue of Warren, AR and nurse practitioner, Janice Sample of Texarkana, AR. They practice whole "person" medicine, exactly what I needed.

My love, admiration and sincerest thank you to my friends and family who had to hold my hand through some really scary scrapes. There are too many of you to name, but you know who you are. No words can capture my gratitude.

CONTENTS

PRELUDE TO JOY

I don't count it a small thing at all that I'm able to write this book. By all medical accounts, I probably should not be here, let alone have the capabilities of writing yet another memoir that details a very personal side of my life, similar to my work in *The Rape of Innocence: Taking Captivity Captive.* And even at the start of this book, as I pour out the contents of my heart, I am awake in pain that is constantly shouting its warning of some dysfunction in my body, pain that hinders my productivity, that disturbs my comfort... yet, it is this very pain that has restored my praise, heightened my own private yearnings for God, and have given me inner fortitude not to be easily undone.

Yes, the tears are falling, but it is not cries of

defeat that come from my mouth. No, no, no! You misunderstand. These tears are the tears of victory cascading down my face reminding me that this precious life is frail like a newborn, sometimes hard, but to be cherished for sure, to be used, every moment to its fullest potential. These tears are the dying away of the old superficial, dare I say materialistic and shallow little girl and the awakening of a woman wholly set on declaring for herself and all sufferers in her reach that THIS too shall pass and WE shall be better for it. This is the awakening of a soldier, one who is fully engaged and well equipped to do what is needed and to deal with whatever comes next. This is the disengagement of my fleshly weaknesses' control over godly freedoms. These tears are the place where the last of misery in its truest sense dies and joy lives.

If you can bear the truth, come with me on this journey, this beautiful walk through the true power of pain.

THE DISEASE INSIDE DISEASE

As a child, health issues were never anything I concerned myself with. I was fairly healthy, rarely even catching a cold. No childhood diseases to speak of. My worst nemesis was the earaches that'd seize me from time to time.

After having two sons at a young age, I made a terrible decision that led to a lifelong struggle, one that also opened the door to other health issues. At the ripe young age of sixteen, I had my second son who died right after I allowed my doctor to tie my tubes. Unheard of now, I know, but not then. At that time, with the birth of two children, I was medically considered an adult, consenting enough to determine my own reproductive future while being wheeled back for an emergency surgery, alone, and terrified out of my mind with all the information they were throwing at me.

Though I'd suffered a broken leg when I was hit by a car the first time, though I'd suffered severe pavement burns after being hit by a car a second time a year after that, nothing prepared me for the suffering I'd see for many years behind that day. I didn't know heartbreak until after that day.

There is a disease that exists inside the very nature of a disease. While disease itself is physical and it attacks and destroys as an enemy sent on a mission, the double whammy of a disease, the disease within the disease, is that it has the uncanny ability to steal our joy, kill our hopes and destroy our faith. So the real enemy of what happens to us daily when we are ill is not the physical, but the destruction of our powerhouse, our inner force to survive, our will to live. The disease inside the disease works away at us daily to make us give up, settle for whatever is happening, or even pray for a swifter end. This disease is a gateway disease, weakening you to everything else that would try to attack you.

The first disease to be diagnosed in my life was anemia. It was so bad with the birth of my second child, in fact, that I had to have a blood transfusion because of blood loss. But I was young. Sickness was new to me. No little disease like anemia would be my undoing. No way!

The second disease to touch my life was infertility and believe me, for a woman, that is a terrible disease. But being young and fresh to the fight, I took even that in stride. I researched, I saved, I worked to have my tubes untied and snatched my fertility back from the child who had once signed it away. I thought I won that fight on the day my wonderful doctor informed me that the procedure was a success. It was the best $5,000 I'd ever spent. I was young, untattered yet. But the battles would get worst.

Another disease, one which had always been there though I had no name for it, was depression. Now some may not call it a disease, but remember what I said diseases do. This battlecat was no different. It was a tough monstrosity of a humdinger. This disease battled with me both night and day. There were no quick fixes and no amount of research or money eased those constant attacks on my mind. Still being fairly young, I made a terrible assumption that this little thing was just a little thing and it'd go away. I underestimated my first real opponent and it nearly cost me my life. Yes, after six full fledge suicide attempts and many other times of plotting and planning, I can honestly say that I did not know what I was dealing with. This monkey would ride my back through every other disease I battled.

The next opponent that boldly approached me was tubal pregnancies, one of which ended with the loss of my best tube with baby entow. Oh yes, death after death of what I wanted the most was not without consequence. That depression monkey grew larger and larger each time I got a bad report. I got so low that I was praying to God to just take me because I could not imagine living with the emotional pain I was feeling. I was dying on the inside. It was like a malignant tumor that ate away at every dream I ever had, that drained away the money I made faster than I could make it, that made me so desperate that I began doing and trying anything to hold on to that dream of being a mother to many children. Depression was starting to show on me and my youth felt like a thing of the past. But even in all this, I had no clue what was coming.

After a brief reprieve and a few bouts with small, powerless nemeses, one of my biggest enemies, one designed seemingly with every weakness I had in its mind, knocked at my door and took me captive. In January 2005, after several months of unexplained illness and then what I thought was a miracle, my fertility doctor discovered only days before I was set to undergo in vitro fertilization that I had hyperthyroidism, or more accurately, Grave's disease. I'd never even heard of it, but it became a part of my daily life.

Being so close to a nearly sure thing with children, and having just spent $15,000 to have all types of pills and injections, and having had 19 fertilized eggs, 9 of which made it to the five day embryo status, I was not about to be undone. So I tried to fight it. After several hospitalizations, a thyroid that was stubborn and didn't want to die was killing me. My heart rate was sky high and all the while my doctor's ominous warning played over and over in my head. This was serious! It could kill me. It was indeed killing me.

I could no longer walk from one end of the house to the other without stopping for a rest. I could no longer skate, play softball, run, talk on the phone and walk simultaneously without sounding like an Olympic runner to the person on the other end. I couldn't even fold a whole load of laundry without being wiped out and needing rest. My whole life was effectively altered.

After years of battling with it, always hoping to be free of it, I finally regained a certain amount of my life back. And just when I thought I might have control back, another hard to diagnose disease made its way into my life. It came on strong and sudden. Blinding headaches, complete loss of sensation on the left side of my body, days of being unable to walk, nights of crying all night long in agony, seizures that left me sometimes on the floor on my face not breathing. At one point, I was diagnosed with meningitis, at another Rocky Mountain Spotted Fever, at another migraines, at another a fainting disorder, and finally I was even diagnosed with epilepsy. Multiple Sclerosis was considered but in truth, my body was being eaten alive by that TKO specialist named lupus. And this is where this book truly begins for me and for my readers.

Before this disease, I'd been fighting the wind, strong-willed at times, wimpy and afraid at others. Before this disease, I'd been so busy feeling like the whole world was against me and that life was just this totally unfair thing I had to live through and hope that God heard enough of my prayers to at least sustain me. Before this disease, I was already an ordained elder, a business owner, an author, a ghetto success story if you will... poor little girl raised on welfare in a dysfunctional home hits it big and finds herself being trusted enough to be a light to others. I was already those things and yet had no idea that I was the biggest fraud of all. It wasn't because I didn't believe what I said could happen. No. My problem was much more personal. I'd been beaten down so much that I no longer believed they could happen to ME.

People praised me for having the answers while I suffered in anguish looking to and awaiting my own answers from God. I was a knowledgeable person who laid biblical theory out that any believer could make work for them, and often did... everybody but me. I was pointing others to the light and all the while too afraid to try to get there again myself.

The disease inside the diseases had me down for the count. Depression wore me out. I was out of there and I didn't care anymore because caring hurt too much. I was tired of pain and would do anything to avoid it. It seemed to me that this last bad boy had won because it was just proof that God cared less than two grapes about me, at least that was my opinion at the time. I had yet to experience true pain or its power, but I was about to and my life would never be the same.

Chapter 1

THE EXPLOSION

An explosion is destructive but not all destruction is a bad thing. When you build up towers of falsehoods for protection, when you wear so many masks that you keep forgetting who you really are, when you hate yourself so much that you don't even bother to want good things anymore, when you have given up on you and built a life around that, then something destructive has to come and tear up all those stays that hold you prisoner.

For me, after what seemed a lifetime of being worn down, of having the foundation chipped at little by little, my walls began to crumble. And because some semblance of control was necessary for me, when I saw that I couldn't control the life I had and turn it into the life I wanted, I shifted and tried to make a home in the life I felt I had no choice but to live miserably. I didn't look miserable on the outside. I didn't sound miserable in my daily interactions, but I was miserable, greatly depressed, all while going to church and reading my Bible. Even that did nothing to help. No amount of sermons I preached or heard did anything to truly turn my sadness around.

WHAT?!!! DID SHE REALLY JUST SAY THAT AND CALL HERSELF A PREACHER?

For me, that was my reality and the horrible fact of it is, I was not alone by any stretch of the imagination. My health issues and the helplessness that came along with them were my explosion. They tore down pride. They tore down my emotional stays. They tore down my goals. They tore me down. Every grand dream I'd ever dared to dream was destroyed by this explosion of healthcare crisis after crisis. I was down, but I was not out. This bad thing was going to turn into a good thing for me even though I didn't know it at the time.

What the world considers bad may be the best thing to happen to us but not for the reasons we wish. What we think we want is a far cry from what we really need most times. For me, sickness taught me things I'd never taken time to learn while I was healthy.

I realized through my oft crises that this was not my world. This world has a master. This is not my final place to walk and thus I'm here only for a time and that time is too short to be wrapped up in my own dreams and desires. I'm chosen and sent. The sacrifice of the job means that it isn't my will that is important to be done. No. If I am to have a Master, a Lord, one that saved me, and if I am to accept Him, then what has to become most important to me is that His will is done in and through me. And that brought on the conflicts within the conflicts in which pain, what I'd considered my mortal enemy, became my best friend.

PAIN POWER

Pain by its very definition is unpleasant feelings, discomfort or downright agony. Now who wants that as a friend? No one. Who wants to experience unpleasant sensations and feelings of discomfort? No one. Who will feel it before leaving this life? Everyone. Since we have to feel it, the key is to figure out what we can about it and how it works.

In nature, the sensation of pain in the body happens when something is wrong with the original design of the body. Whether internal or external, signals are sent to the brain to say, "Houston, we have a problem! There's something going on that requires your immediate attention." Things are no different in the spirit of pain. Pain is there as an alert system to warn us of a problem. While most people think a little pain pill can fix that "problem", the only thing that pill can actually do is quieten the alarm system. That pill turns off your alert telling you something is wrong. Day after day, you are pushing these pills down to drown out that constant beeping, ringing, buzzing of alarm, but all you've really accomplished is to allow whatever is setting off that alarm to grow and further infect your internal controls without detection.

While I was going through chronic pain, I had to face so many issues, both childhood and current fears. I remembered how my mother became a drug addict- being shot by her husband and becoming addicted to strong pain medications. I was terrified of becoming addicted to pain meds. I would lie in bed and hurt for hours, crying, shaking and rocking, trying not to take a pill. I'd try to do anything to distract myself, including a lot of horrible writing. I wanted to master my pain, bring it under subjection to the strength of my mind. I tried to think myself happy, think myself strong, think myself healed, but my redemption from pain was not to be found in my mind, at least not in that way.

One night during prayer, it came to me so quietly. It was as if a voice whispered, "Pain is not your problem, child. Pain is only alerting you to the presence of a problem."

I sat there bewildered by that. I'd tried getting answers from doctors to no avail, and to be fair to them, they are not the creators of the body, so they only know the bits they know. We cannot expect them to have all our answers as complex as the body is. So I asked God to teach me. I wanted to get out of the situation, but that was not the lesson He'd prepared for me. Rather, the lesson was to understand the intricate workings of the body and how it correlates to the spiritual world and all healings, whether physical, emotional, or mental.

You see, we are people who hate feeling anything unpleasant and many of us are shallow by nature. We don't naturally like to think of the whys in life. We only want the situation handled and the discomfort ended as soon as possible. We judge things on a superficial level. If we see apples on a tree, we call it a good apple tree because it produces apples. It is mature, we think. But the maker of the tree, and thus the apples, judges deeper. Is this apple sweet as it should be? Is this apple as big as it could be? Is the color right? Does this tree need more fertilizer? More water? More sunshine? We don't see that deeply. We don't know that deeply. We only know what we want and expect. We are willing to sell out sometimes to get the easy answers and quick fixes that fix nothing. How sad!

The first lesson I had to learn in my chronic pain was that pain was my body's way of crying out for some attention and help. I needed to do something differently, to either stop doing something or start doing something. It was missing something. It needed me to pay attention to my actions, my thoughts, my words. There was a disagreement somewhere among my body members.

I wrote down all the things my body was no longer getting that it got plenty of when I was healthy. I was no longer exercising. I didn't drink water. I didn't even try to eat right. I was stressed, depressed and frustrated all the time. Even my prayer life was weak. Oh, it was strong for others, but when it concerned me, I'd been beaten down to the place where all I could ask for was God to have mercy on me. I looked at my life and I was doing everything wrong and completely ignoring the bits about health that I already knew. No vitamins or minerals were being supplemented to my diet. I had been asking for this trouble for a long time.

The explosion of health crises had finally gotten my attention. This temple that God gave me had certain requirements, none of which we can say we are unable to fulfill because God supplies all of our needs according to His riches in glory. There's no good thing we'll ever lack. He is thoughtful of us, constantly giving and surrounding us in love and provision. But here I was hitting a brick wall and trapped in the back by a mountain. It wasn't moving by prayer and fasting or any of the things I thought would work. It wasn't responding to my cries, my medications or my willpower. It was there and would remain there until I got up and did something different, something necessary which was to give my temple the care it required.

An explosion is impossible to ignore, which is why God allows them in our lives. Sometimes, we simply do not listen to that still small voice of His. We do not heed what we read in the Bible. We do not truly tune in to the information God has given others because at first, we don't see the need, and later we don't see how it can help us in light of the damage done. We are stubborn at all the wrong times and weak-willed when we shouldn't be. We don't sleep how and when we should. We don't eat when and what we should. We don't move as much and how we should, but we expect everything to work on our behalf. We expect these bodies to take our abuse and function anyway. We expect our bodies not to complain if they lack oxygen, water, nourishment, rest or peace. We ignore some things because they are weird, some things because they are new, other things because they are old, other things because they are too difficult and many things because they are too easy. Hence now, we are laid up in bed, putting on more weight, popping pills to stop the agony of chronic pain and wondering where we went wrong.

Am I saying that only those who abuse their bodies are ill? No. Some illnesses we are born with and there's not much we can do but use our faith to live the best life possible. Some illnesses come despite our best efforts to supply care for our bodies, but this chapter isn't for those who have done everything right just to find sickness at the other end. This particular chapter is for those who, like me, thought that we had time to get all that care stuff right later. We were too busy to even pay ourselves any attention. We lived those high stress lifestyles and got caught in mid-stride by illness and pain. But hang on and keep reading because I'm sure I'm about to introduce a chapter just for you.

Chapter 2
STUBBORN RECOGNITION

As I went from doctor to doctor, seeking to figure out what was wrong with me, I found out that naming an illness was not an exact science. While some diseases were easy to spot, others played possum, hid behind vague symptoms and generally were masters of disguise. Lupus was one of those master-of-disguise diseases. The symptoms of it were shared by so many other illnesses in the beginning. By the time the more pronounced symptoms showed up, the illness had been present for some time causing serious problems and damage.

When I found out that I had lupus, another autoimmune disorder, I felt lost and hopeless. I felt like my body had tuned in to those times when I was suicidal, depressed and full of self-hatred, but hadn't gotten the message that those days were now over. Like Grave's disease and alopecia, something else that I'd had happen a few times before, my body was attacking itself. It was confused as to what should and shouldn't be here or there. It was fighting when there was no battle to fight. How do you defeat yourself to keep yourself from killing you? That was the question I pondered over and over. I was killing myself, now successfully, when I didn't really want to die. I wanted to live. I wanted a full life. I wanted to keep writing, keep speaking, keep preaching, keep helping others, keep waking up everyday looking at my family. I wanted more children. I had a lot of life left in me. Why? Why was this happening now?

Now right here is where I take a sidebar to tell you something most doctors won't. By the time your body begins crying for help loud enough for you to hear and do something about it, some damage has already been done. I'd had Grave's at least a full year before it was diagnosed. Apparently, it was the same with lupus. My body had been without basic necessities so long that it was confused. It had read all of those negative emotions that I grew up on, fostered into adulthood and fed upon for most of my life. It had interpreted my will and the process of premature death had begun long ago. I hated me so much that I did whatever I wanted to do to me whenever I got ready.

I didn't like water so I didn't drink it and I didn't care how many times I became dehydrated. If I wanted to eat at midnight, I was a stick so I'd eat what and whenever I dang well pleased. So what about the constant bellyaches I had. I'd pop a Tums or Rolaids and keep it moving. When I cooked, I loved salt, plenty of it. In fact, I liked salt so much, I ate it out of my hand. That was ME. I'd done all this amazing damage to myself when I just didn't care about my future, when I felt invincible. But lo and behold, what I started then was affecting me now. What could I do?

I didn't know what to do, but I knew what I would not do. I would no longer allow negative emotions to live in me, confusing my body and mind. I would not give up hope that I might be free from all of it one day, totally free, without medications and without fear of the disease coming back. I would not blame God as if He'd willed some big bad horrible disease on me and expected me to deal with it the best way I knew how. I would not blame my past, family, the devil, or anyone. When we start playing the blame game, we take our energy and put it into something empty of power. I knew I was not going to do the negativity thing. That was the majority of my problem. After figuring out all that I wouldn't do, it by default told me a few things I'd have to do.

I had to tap into true joy and remain joyful, no matter how bad the pain got. I had to trust God, even though this was a problem I'd created. I had to focus on loving HIM and loving myself. I had to make sure I focused on forgiving those who'd wronged me and forgiving myself for my own ignorance and wrongs. Ultimately, I had to pay closer attention to me, taking better care of my body. I didn't know how this new attitude would help my broken body, but I knew it definitely couldn't hurt. I wanted to enjoy the life left in me even if I had to enjoy it from my bed most days, or through the internet, or through the fog of medications.

I was suffering from intolerance of heat and cold, fast heart rate, unstable blood pressure, severe headaches, partial blindness, left side numbness and weakness, a noticeable limp when I was able to get out of the bed, severe dizziness, constant drowsiness, unannounced seizures, unannounced spasms, bladder issues, constant hallucinations so that I was diagnosed with schizophrenia, and quick weight gain. I was a huge ball of crazy symptoms and finding some kind of joy or happiness in the midst of it would be a challenge but not one without its rewards.

The fighter in me at first was loath to even accept the diagnosis. I hate when someone gives me some "nothing I can do about it" news. It always makes me want to say, "Who me? Watch me, then. I bet I'll do something about it." But this time, it wasn't my fight, at least not in that way. It wasn't for me to go trying to bulldoze my way through this illness and trying to force it into remission by all means necessary. Nope, not this time. But that stubborn side of me, that side that had gotten everything the hard way, wanted to protest. It wanted to fight, wanted to complain, wanted to muster up every believer with even half of a prayer life to try to force God's hand. My stubborn side didn't want to do what something on the inside of me knew I'd have to do at some point. It didn't want to calm down and accept God and the fullness of who He was even if that meant no healing would come. I didn't understand that sometimes, giving up the fight is the only way to win it. I didn't understand that this time, this disease, wouldn't respond to that bulldozer mentality. This one would only respond to the power of God and the power of love, me loving God, loving myself and loving others. So stubbornly at first, I came to recognize the source of all my medical woes- ME. It was the lifestyle I'd lived, the emotions I'd allowed in, and the way I'd ignored the bigger part of who God was. Stubbornly at first, I had to recognize that I am not strong enough to overcome this one, not this time. I had only enough strength left to fall upon my face in submission to God and ask HIM to teach me how to live this life. I'd made a terrible mess of things, done nearly everything wrong, destroyed myself. I was as dead as they come. I needed life and I was no life-giver. I needed God in a way I'd never realized I needed HIM before.

Chapter 3
WHERE DO I FIND GOD?

Coming to the conclusion that I need God was the easy part. Reconnecting with Him much more difficult, not because of Him but because of the state I was in. I was trying to "find" God, but God was never lost, and had not departed. Thus, again I was spinning my wheels. I was looking outside of myself for an answer that would only come through making peace between myself and God, from an inside job.

Right after I began going through repeated hospitalizations and E.R. visits, I began to lose faith. It began to feel like this illness would always be in my life and I'd always be miserably sick and barely able to function. And so, even before the doctors began to give up, I'd given up. I was praying for death and release versus healing and restoration for a time. While my whole church family labored in prayer for me to be healed, I was so broken and confused by pain that I was in direct opposition to those prayers. I wanted only for it to end.

While not preaching or trying to convert anyone in this book, I find it necessary to talk about the role of faith and speech in healing and wholeness. I remember something my Physical Science teacher used to say in school. "Just because you can't see gravity or don't believe in it doesn't exempt you from the effects of it (gravity)." In the same way, whether or not we believe in God does not change the fact that He exists and He is Most Powerful. Often, when people are diagnosed with chronic illnesses, either they cling to God more desperately or reject Him more definitely. But either way, most sick people have very strong feelings about faith, a case for it or against it. And the list of people proclaiming supernatural healing grows by the hundreds or thousands each day. Yet, growing as rapidly are those who became disillusioned because they were diagnosed with a disease. In their minds, their faith should have protected them from ever becoming ill. They feel that God has failed them and allowed some awful evil to come into their lives by way of sickness and disease. And so, they create a horrible cycle, speaking negative words with worsening results until it culminates into some form of death. And since they blame God, they will not turn to Him, the solution.

Whatever condition you are in spiritually will create either a circle of blessing, healing and wholeness or a circle of loss, destruction and depression. Fortunately, God isn't like mankind. He is easily entreated. He doesn't hold grudges or anger. He doesn't hold the past over our heads. He doesn't hide away. He presents Himself moment by moment as a real option in our lives. Though He's never in need of finding, He still must be sought.

There are those, who in false humility, assume they cannot wait until everything falls apart to run to God. Guilt won't allow them. They ascribe to God humanly characteristics like pettiness and cruelty, mockery and grudges. They believe God won't hear them when they know they need Him most, but it does not matter what has transpired in the past, God has made Himself available to all at any time through prayer. This all may seem like a long detour, but bear with me because I had to make those prior points to get to the meat of this chapter.

When I became ill, I was in a sinful relationship. I was separated from my godly husband and making plans to marry another man. I was in adultery. I was shacking. I was lying. I wasn't faithful at church. I was backslidden. I was depressed. And in that low place, though I knew God and had previously preached the Gospel, I felt completely alienated from Him. I didn't know how to boldly approach the throne of grace to find help in troubling times. I didn't know how to accept His goodness or grace. I didn't feel that He was with me or for me. I felt like I was an enemy to God and thus, I was rendered powerless to believe the scriptures applied to me too, that I could be healed too.

Healing is often applied to the heart, as in restoring broken hearts. It is also applied to the body, restoring health. But healing is an all-inclusive package. And often, the reason many of us do not walk in better health is because we hadn't accepted the fullness of healing and health into our lives. We hadn't allowed our minds to be healed and purged and of every contrary thing. We hadn't allowed our hearts to mend from every break and tear. We hadn't allowed our spirits to mend through prayer and meditation. And even now, some of you are reading this thinking that all of that sounds like a long process that you don't have time to indulge. Again, you are short-changing yourself to make time for the things that destroy rather than accepting healing.

When your body has been attacked with viruses, bacteria, or when it chooses to attack itself, you are in need of healing. You can't go and do all that everyone else goes and does. You have to sit down. Get quiet. Listen. Make amends and corrections. You cannot afford to live haphazardly, taking chances with your physical, mental and spiritual wellness. And make no mistake about it, you are a whole with many parts, but if you don't apply healing to all of you, you only buy time until the next calamity.

If you think of life in terms of giving and receiving, everything we have, including illness, is given to us. But in that transaction of giving and receiving, you also have the option not to receive. You can deny a "gift" just as easily as you can accept it. There are times when we begin to claim things that we know we don't want. The world's language system is set up to make sure you own various diagnoses. The doctor says, "You have lupus." and you immediately go home and inform family and friends. You say, "I have lupus." And so, in the end, you truly do have lupus and each time you say it, you're making it stronger in your life. You are making a verbal commitment to something you truly do not want to possess.

Sometimes, like in my case, a disease may be your reality. There is diabetes or cancer or lupus in your body. That is real. It is fact. But it isn't the truth of you so you don't have to accept it as a personal truth. You don't have to allot a permanent space to it in your life. In fact, I truly believe that no disease is permanent and that our bodies can heal itself from practically anything, but it happens as a result of wholeness, not embracing the disease but embracing yourself. The fight is to not lose yourself in the onslaught of body attacks.

Dealing with a chronic illness that brings a lot of pain and discomfort can cause disorientation. We receive disease in our bodies and start to doubt our own healing abilities. We trust too much in statistics and not enough in the bodies we've been living in all our lives. We abandon our bodies, and so in a strange way, we abandon ourselves.

Chapter 4
GOD IN MY WORDS

When I first began having seizures, there was so much embarrassment. I'd seen my mom and grandmother go through grand mal and petite mal seizures. I didn't want that family heirloom. I hated the violent shakes, tongue biting, and all the other less than desirable side effects of a seizure. But there I was, suddenly having epileptic attacks. And in the beginning, I laid down and took it. I didn't truly understand what was happening so I prayed for healing. I didn't understand how to take dominion over my body and call it back into alignment. In fact, it was the seizures that taught me the lesson of using my words to find healing.

After about a year, I began reading all that I could find about seizures, what caused them and what happens when they occur. Come to find out, it is a rapid increase of the electrical activity in your brain. That surge causes the brain to send out impulses which in turn causes the nerves to have a reaction, which appears as violent, uncontrolled shaking in epilepsy. Basically, it's a miscommunication between brain and body. I heard a nurse once say that it is the brain going spastic and saying way too much too swiftly for the nerves to interpret. Either way, armed with knowledge, I was able to direct my prayers and my words to call my body back into alignment when I began to slip into an aura.

Sure enough, with targeted prayer and speech, my faith became targeted and I noticed the difference almost immediately. Several seizures I would have had didn't happen and to be honest, it soon got to a place where the only time I'd have any seizures was when I was too busy and stressed to pick up my body's subtle clues. Still, I learned to call balance to my life and I saw a rapid decrease of seizures.

During another low point with the lupus, I was required to use a walker because of the weakness and numbness on my left side. I was still a newlywed and had a young, vibrant husband. I didn't want to follow him around pushing a walker. I didn't want to be some old, sick burden of a wife to him. But between the illnesses and the bad calls in medication, I didn't have a choice. I was in the thick of several chronic illnesses and it was deeper than thinking myself better. It would require much more than mind over matter to heal. Luckily, I met a doctor as a friend and he was the first to diagnose me with lupus. He told me the ins and outs of the disease and asked me a simple question. "Do you want to walk normally again? It's going to hurt." Well, of course I did. Why would I want to be in my thirties on a walker? I didn't care how much it hurt.

For a couple of weeks, this man had me doing squats, walking up and down stairs, and generally doing every painful exercise I could have imagined to get my body back in line. Every joint that had stiffened and swollen in those past months of inactivity were being exercised. Gritting through the pain of it all, I had to pray through the workouts. I had to pray through the pain, and pray for sleep when my whole body ached. But in less than a month, I no longer needed the walker. In less than three months, I no longer had to drag my left leg behind me. And in less than six months, my range of motion improved so much that I was performing better than I had in the days before I became ill.

Through those two things, I realized that we are soul, spirit and body. We must use our entire arsenal to keep those in alignment. Our thoughts, words and deeds must also be in alignment. We cannot do the right deeds with the wrong thoughts and words and expect a true healing. Somehow, if we are to give ourselves a fighting chance, we must learn how to keep balance, and words spoken aloud have a tremendous ability to guide our thoughts which guide our actions. Could it be, God uses our words? Indeed, He empowered our words. Use them wisely in your fight against illness.

Chapter 5
CRY ME A RIVER

It is amazing how powerful tears are, but at times, they feel rather useless. When you know God as Father, sometimes you want Him to be like a human father whose heart is moved by your tears, so much so that He will turn away pain and every wicked thing that comes to bring you anguish of heart. Both fortunately and unfortunately, God is not like a human father. While your tears will not change His will, that doesn't mean He isn't moved by them. For sure, His heart melts with the anguish of our hearts and bodies. But His plan is eternal and His work is beyond perfect. He knows what's best.

Nevertheless, the Bible records that God bottles every one of our tears. And surely, if He is taking up time to bottle the tears, He also knows the meaning of every single one of them. He knows what pain or what joy created them all. I mean seriously, God is intimately involved with our lives. He isn't an absentee father or deadbeat dad. He is right there every moment watching over His most prized possession- His creation.

I remember when I was at my lowest point. I was ill, broke and facing legal problems. I didn't know which way to go or what to do. It felt as if the walls of life were closing in on me. I became despondent. I was worried all the time. Stress was making the medication I was prescribed practically useless. I was unable to perform my wifely duties and my husband was beginning to complain. My son was tired. I was tired. It had all taken a toll.

One day while home alone, I broke down and began to cry. At first, it was because of the overwhelming pressure and then because of the overwhelming sadness. I felt sorry for myself. I wanted God to feel sorry for me, see my pain, change something, release me from all the suffering. And for a time, I prayed that He'd even take my life. I didn't want it anymore. I didn't want to struggle forever, hide forever, keep living with my past blocking the view of a promising future I'd glimpsed. I cried so long that I ran out of tears and energy. Finally, after long and exhausting sobs, I fell asleep. And I discovered something important about crying, something that I'm going to share for the first time ever in this book.

The purpose of tears is not to change your life or your situation or God's mind about His will. The purpose of tears is to cleanse us emotionally, to open us up and expose us to the purest form of personal truth. I understand that many people fake tears, but at this moment, we're discussing the true emotional upheavals that come up in our lives. Those times are the most precious and powerful times of our lives, even if we don't recognize it as such during those moments.

When you break and the tears come without permission, you are experiencing a moment that is free of facades, lies and judgment. At that moment of desperation, you are free from all the masks. Tears represent full exposure, an emotional nudity that empowers you to change. No doubt, the water from our souls is sometimes the only thing strong enough to pierce through the layers of masks we wear. It is then that God can deal with the naked you because at that point, you're as free to be you as you were when you were an infant. Tears represent freedom and can lead to a wholeness that is unbelievable. Tears can lead you to peace. They can lead you to joy. And while you may not feel like it as you lie down upon your pillow and cry yourself a river, God is attending to every wet drop that falls from your face. He is interpreting them and bottling them for the day that He will reward your life.

I remember being hospitalized for schizophrenia once. I was having hallucinations and talking to people who weren't actually there. And in the midst of it, I had a moment of clarity. And I thought, how can someone else interpret my reality? I see my grandmother. She's speaking to me and I am speaking to her. I see these things and thereby, they are real to me. And I began to question our entire human understanding of this world. How can I have a conversation with a dead person, or see animals that aren't there? How can my mind concoct what isn't real to anyone else?

It was a pickle that I was in. The morning after I was admitted, I woke up alone. My husband was gone to work. The hallucinations were over. All that was left was the shame of having doctors ask me a thousand psychological questions. As I was explaining more about the sexual abuse that had nothing to do with the hallucinations, the random thought came to me - cry me a river. My life sounded messed up trying to explain it to someone else. I sounded unstable, emotionally needy and aloft at the same time. The people in my life sounded uncaring. It was just a mess. But the thought kept coming, "cry me a river".

Later as I began to pray, I thought about all the water references in the Bible. And clarity hit me. God builds rivers with our tears, rivers that flow in and out of our hearts and lives. Only He can navigate it, but our tears are a conduit for Him to operate through. Our blessed and loving Father didn't waste a thing when building us. All things truly do work together for our good and His glory. How wonderful to realize, even the

worst parts of our lives have a purpose and that
it is good.

Chapter 6
STRESS THAT...

In any illness, doctors find some medication or other to prescribe. Sometimes, it is only for symptoms and sometimes it is actually for correction of the problem. Either way, there seems to be a medicine for everything except the number one killer of all time- stress! And what is stress, exactly? Where does it come from and what can cure it?

Traditionally, stress is defined as strain caused by anxiety or overwork. That's an understatement. Stress is the result of trying to control what is not yours to control, trying to change what you're unable to change, or trying to be who you were not created to be. Stress is caused by getting ahead of God, or lagging too far behind. Stress is caused by not taking time to appreciate and love self. Stress is caused by skewed perspective. This list could go on but to sum it up, stress happens when God slips away from first place in our lives, when we stop obeying and begin trying to figure it all out on our own. Stress is a direct result of wavering faith. And the cure? A medicated soul.

In the beginning of my battle, I kept looking for natural solutions to my problems. Even though I was a well-known and respected minister of the Gospel, I was approaching my issue from a human only perspective. I wanted a real, physical healing, but I wasn't seeing the spiritual issues. I didn't see the issues of sin in my life. I didn't see the issues of iniquity in my heart. I didn't see the doubt and distrust in the beginning. I only saw the problem and the outcome I desired. Hence, my original approach made the problem worse rather than better. I had a lot to learn.

While I have no intentions of preaching to anyone in this book, there are some things that cannot be said enough. One of those things have to do with the fact that God did not create our bodies to die or to sin. He created them for goodness and favor to flow through them for an eternity. The creation and design didn't change. So what did? Us. We opened the door for sin and iniquity and that brought in disease and distress. After Adam and Eve's fall, all other humans inherited sin as the primary disease, not of the body, but of the soul. We're born in a bad way, even if we don't feel it until later on in life. Yes, sin is the cause of every imperfection because there was no flaw in the original design, unless you want to consider freedom of choice a flaw. Personally, I consider it the best gift available. God gave freedom to us as a gift. And the heart of His plan for our lives is based upon our decision to either love and obey Him or not.

Every decision to disobey, every decision to ignore the truth, every time we relegate God to a secondary position, all of those choices have consequences. Stress is a sin-related killer. How can I say that? Because the proof is evident.

Stress is a direct result of worry, which is sin; anxiety, which is sin; disobedience, which is sin;

or pride, which is also sin. No matter how many books I write on the subject, I must stress the fact that sin has both spiritual and natural consequences. Many of the autoimmune disorders, like Lupus and Fibromyalgia, are caused primarily by stress. It causes the body to wig out and become unable to distinguish the good from the bad. Huh. Sounds just like what happens to us mentally when we engage in sin too long. Our conscience is seared and we become unable to distinguish right from wrong. As I stated previously, the proof is all there for anyone to piece together.

My personal battle with stress was fueled by the control freak that lived inside me. I felt compelled to control everything that I was connected to or cared about because I'd been hurt by others frequently. Regardless, I grew up battling depression caused from sexual abuse and a broken home. The normal stress children felt was not mine. Tests and studying never stressed me. It wasn't even cause for a second thought most times. My stressors were sexual abuse, alcoholism and drug use in my family, poverty, the care of my grandmother, the care of a baby, and lack of positive companionship. As an adult, the stress was worsened by the many responsibilities I had. Eventually, it was so bad that I didn't know how to appreciate the good times and the peaceful days. It always felt like something was wrong when I did get a moment to rest or a time of peace and quiet.

I remember the day I sat down and began to be proactive about the diseases that were attacking my body. I started with research. I wanted to know the origin of the problems I was having. Every single one (Grave's disease, fibro, lupus and epilepsy) was either caused by and/or worsened by stress. In my case personally with late onset of epilepsy, all of my diseases were caused by my high intensity lifestyle. The type A personality I'd always been proud of had backfired on me. To make it plain, I was killing myself. That revelation rocked me back on my heels. All those years of suicidal thoughts and attempts, all of the self-hatred, all of the depression from my past had culminated into an event that would either make me or break me. Personally, I refuse to be broken unless it is by divine will of our heavenly Father. Circumstances shake me, hurt me and yes, I experience trauma. But my brokenness is reserved for God.

I had to make some decisions. I had to heal and I knew that healing would have to begin in my soul.

Chapter 7
THE MEDICATED SOUL

The soul is a complexity in a sin-shattered world. In the original design, there was no sin. So having a mind full of imagination and intellect, having a will, and having emotions were the biggest blessing. They allow for each individual person to experience God and His miraculous work in very personal ways. Alas, when sin entered the picture, our greatest gifts became mixed blessings at best, a curse at the worst.

After all the research I did, after all the faithless prayers, after all the medicating my body, the emptiness would not leave. Neither would the diseases. At first, it seemed that the last drop of my faith had failed me. I pondered whether I deserved to hurt, to suffer, or if maybe God was angry with me. My soul was full of anguish. There was no rest for me. My mind, my body and my emotions were in constant upheaval. But I kept thinking, "There must be a way through this. Things can't always be this way."

Our bodies were created from dirt and will return to the dirt. They decay and fall apart and become one with the earth again. Our spirits were God-breathed into us. That part belongs to Him. But our souls are uniquely ours. We can medicate the body but it will not change the fact that decay begins as soon as growth ends. However, when we medicate the soul, we are providing ourselves with eternal benefits. So how do you medicate the soul? You feed it to align it with the Spirit of God. It is the Spirit that brings healing, wholeness and seals us for redemption.

Think of your soul as a person without a body. It is your intangible person. Your mind is about how you think, how you process information. It is composed of the intellect (factual, logical, grounded, learned side) and the imagination (free, creative, mutable side). If the mind is not guided, it can lead us into places we do not need to be. The mind cannot be left to simply exist. No. No. No! We must be diligent to guard what we see and hear, which will directly affect how we think.

The will is all about want and purpose. A person cannot touch or handle your purpose and desires, but they are real and powerful nonetheless. We must guide our will. We cannot be ungrounded when it comes to our desires and the purposes of our hearts.

The emotions are probably the most discussed but the least understood. It's about feeling and sensation, but also inner energy. This too must be guided. For some, their faith began through their emotions. And that is a huge problem, to rest our faith on the most fickle part of our make-up.

The soul is influenced by childhood experiences and atmosphere even when we do not remember them outright. And unfortunately, oftentimes for those without God-believing families, that influence is not godly. So as believing adults, we must begin to retrain our souls, guide it through the Word of God so that our mind has a focus, our will has an eternal purpose and so that our emotions have a safe place of existence.

Matthew 22: 37 says, *"Jesus said unto him, Thou shalt love the Lord thy God with all thy heart, and with all thy soul, and with all thy mind."* That is the beginning of wholeness. Indeed, the love of God and love for God has the power to mend anything. Yes, I said ANYTHING.

Chapter 8
LESS IS MORE

When you're diagnosed with a chronic, lifelong illness, life changes. How you feel changes. How you think changes. What you desire changes. Sickness is one of the great equalizers. There is no race, no socioeconomic status, no amount of success or recognition that can save you from a chronic illness. What has no cure has no cure for us all. What hurts also hurts for us all. To a chronically ill person, healing and relief is all that matters.

When you're truly sick, all the excess of life falls away out of necessity. How you live becomes more important than where, how you feel becomes more important than what you have. That is probably the best part of illness, learning what you truly don't need. It would be a huge blessing if we could have that freedom without becoming ill because I venture a guess that over half of the diseases that destroy us wouldn't exist if we were not in a hurry to have more and be more. When you are diagnosed with a disease that doctors say will be with you for the rest of your life and shorten your life, all of a sudden, you realize that all that crap that glitters doesn't seem to matter anymore. All that matters is love, family and purpose. Your soul matters.

I remember how low I felt when we began losing things because I was unable to work. Dealing with the wide range of symptoms I was required to deal with had me at a terrible disadvantage. As things began to fall away and our spending power dwindled, I realized how unnecessary most of the things I'd worked to attain truly were. I wasn't less of a woman because I had to drive a beat up old car, walk or catch a ride. Without the French style home with hardwood floors throughout, I was still me. I didn't need all the name brands. My son didn't need it. My husband didn't need it. Those things had been distractions because I had just as many good times without them as I did with them. Sure they were nice, but not worth killing myself over by working long, grueling hours.

In illness, I discovered a mystery of life. Less is more. It doesn't take more money or more possessions to enjoy life. If your heart is ungrateful, no amount of money or possessions will truly fulfill you. You enter into a cycle that will kill you. But when you are grateful and truly take time to experience life for the miracle that it is, you realize that the quality of life is in the moments you share with your loved ones. Quality of life is about making the most of what is given. I'm not saying don't stretch yourself or reach for greatness. In fact, it is just as stressful not to reach for the greatness already inside of you as it is to overextend yourself. The key- balance!

Chapter 9

HEART DISEASE

It's safe to classify sin as a condition. In fact, it is the cause of all disease. But specifically, sin affects the heart. In fact, often that is the opening.

The heart is like a storage facility for all that happens in life. Every good and bad thing affects the heart. The heart plays a role in how the mind processes information. The Bible even tells us that out of the heart flows the issues of life. We're ordered to guard our hearts with all diligence. Then, we're told that the heart is deceptive, but later encouraged that even when our own hearts condemn us, God is greater than our hearts and will set us free. (insert actual scriptures)

To be free of any disease, we must clean our

hearts. We must allow God complete freedom to mold our hearts and remove all dirt and debris. We must open ourselves up to God, trusting Him fully. Only God can truly cure heart disease.

Growing up, I rarely felt loved enough. My father wasn't there and my mother was suffering with her own problems. Raising me fell to my grandmother who gladly took me on. And though I'm sure my parents loved me as much as my grandmother, I didn't see that growing up. I could only feel their absence. It didn't matter how much love my grandmother gave me, the fact that my own parents were not raising me made me feel abandoned. For those who read my first international release, *The Rape of Innocence: Taking Capitivity Captive*, you have already heard the story of my childhood trauma. Suffice to say, I had a lot of holes in my heart by the time I became an adult. I needed healing but I didn't know it right off. I didn't realize that depression was a symptom of heart "dis-ease".

The sadness that saturated my life seemed like it would never end. Because of that sadness,

I didn't eat right. I didn't work out. I didn't care much what I did because none of it seemed to ultimately matter. Even after the initial joy of my salvation, the sadness came right back. Don't crucify me for saying so. Simply accepting Christ didn't automatically fix everything in my life. Christ was my answer, but it took a lot of time to learn how to apply that answer to each situation properly.

In church circles, so often we give the impression that at the point of salvation, everything fixes itself and if not, there is something wrong with you. That's not true. Salvation is the beginning of a lifelong process. There's nothing wrong with you if your life is not perfect the moment you confess Christ as Lord. Fact is, the hard part is reprogramming. Your whole train of thought and way of life must change and that does not happen overnight for anyone. Even Jesus had to have a time of preparation and He was a perfect man and divinity. Let's be real with ourselves and each other. It takes time and knowledge.

Heart dis-ease is rampant and the effects are

obvious, especially in the church. So many people confess coming in and going out hopeless. They are seeking an instant answer, but God seeks to educate us and prepare us for the next life, which is not done instantly.

Chapter 10

THE DEEPER ISSUES

The purpose of this book, as you may have already discovered, is not as much about the physical issue as it is the emotional issues that can cause the physical issues. It is true that there are natural ways to cope with any illness. We have to take care of the physical body. We need to eat right and exercise. We must avoid unnecessary stressors and learn to deal with everyday stress. We must keep our bodies nourished with vitamins and minerals. Those things are evident in our modern society. There are tons of books, millions if not billions of articles about the subject. I stand behind all that has been done to prove the importance of maintenance on these bodies that house us. But there again is the issue- these bodies are only homes for who we are.

To be truly healed and come to terms with physical illness, we must deal with ourselves first. For every illness that has its beginning in neglect, the problem cannot be solved with medication alone. The issue of self-abuse must first be dealt with.

As I shared previously, I was chronically depressed. I was suicidal a great deal of my life, including the majority of my teen and young adult years. I basically hated myself. I abused myself. And even when not consciously trying to, the negative energy that radiated from my soul permeated my body and had dire effects.

Once during my illness, the doctor diagnosed pseudo seizures. Basically, he thought that either I was purposely faking seizures or my subconscious was causing them. It was the strangest feeling to be interviewed about my life again, looking for a trigger for my epileptic events. For awhile, even I thought maybe the seizures weren't real. But then a new wave hit me and finally after being plugged to a machine and housed in a room with a camera, I had a seizure, one so intense that I nearly bit through my tongue and actually wet myself. This isn't something I can discuss without a great deal of shame, but it is necessary for all to see how deeply chronic illness can impact your life.

Afterwards, doctors had a hard time controlling the seizures I had. Dilantin worked, but I had allergic reactions to it, including hives, itching, ringing ears, hallucinations, and more. In the place of that one pill, three had to be added (Keppra, Tegretol and Neurontin). While going through this long, drawn out process and suffering from strong, often painful, exhausting seizures, I had time to reflect. I reflected on what seizures feel like, what they are and how it was affecting me. I began to ask myself questions and deal with the hard answers. Truth was, my mind and my body were not in agreement. Remember, the mind is a facet of the soul, the person that I am. The body is a temple, a house for my soul. So the essence of who I was did not agree with the place I occupied. Gosh, every time I share that revelation, I become goosy. It was so freeing to understand what was going on in my body was also going on in my life, in the spirit realm. That knowledge put me on the path to true and lasting healing.

God's design for existence is cohesion. All things affect all other things so that none of us will ever find satisfaction or fulfillment without each other and without harmony with the will of God. Put simply, all things are connected. When my lifestyle is out of sync with the creation I was destined to be, everything else goes awry also. When my soul wills to do something contrary to God's plan and places my body in disobedience, my spirit cries out. The life force that is within me is hindered from refreshing the temple. Basically, sin interrupts my life energy. The process of renewal is interrupted. And it shows up in different ways in different people.

The above argument is compelling but let me complete it with scriptural reference. Several times in New Testament scriptures, Jesus made reference to the forgiveness of sin and healing as being partners together. Both in the book of James as well as through some of the recountings of the Gospel books, a dynamic case is made for the reality of healing and forgiveness. It is as if God is letting us know that sickness itself is not the problem but rather a symptom of the problem. Sickness is a direct result of the fall from grace and the entrance of sin into the world. Thus to get free and stay free from sickness, we must solve our sin problem and the only way to do so is through Jesus Christ. Now, I made a promise earlier not to preach and I won't, but allow me to finish this thought to prepare you to understand my next few points.

We all know good people who died young, god-fearing people who suffered a long time with some disease, and bad people who lived a long and healthy life. However, from my perspective of illness, lack of physical issues do not mean health just as the presence of physical issues do not necessarily mean illness. What I'm saying is that this book is about unveiling the spiritual realm of health and wholeness and opening ourselves up to understand God's plan in creation and in redemption.

During my years of nearly falling to Grave's

disease, then the addition of Lupus, fibromyalgia and epilepsy, I had to learn how to possess my body again. For all intents and purposes, disease had seized me and taken control. I was a slave to illness and pain. My life was dictated by doctors, nurses, medications and excruciating physical sensations. And honestly, it was nothing doctors did to put me on the road to healthy living. It was the Holy Spirit that led me to delve deeper into my own psyche and understand how I'd been infiltrated in the first place. It was God's gentle hand leading me to a well of living waters in His Word that began the healing process.

At the writing of this book, I'm not disease free from a medical standpoint. However, I have my life back and dominion over this house God gave me for the duration of my stay upon earth. I'm whole and that truth does not change even when pain does come to challenge it, or symptoms flare up to make me doubt. I've learned that even sickness can be a blessing, leading us places we would have never had the strength to go as healthy individuals. For me, sickness in my body kept my soul in check. I am reminded of Paul's thorn in his flesh (insert scripture) and Sarah's conception problem, etc. Not one person in the Bible, rather we see them as major players or minor league, not one of them were without challenges, either physically, mentally, emotionally or usually all three.

Now, all of what I said above is really about this next sentence. Illness can serve several purposes: correction and glory come to mind first. Do you remember reading the recount of when the disciples wondered who'd sinned to cause the man in question to be born blind? Isn't that always the first response to failure, illness or trials? Seems people are more concerned with what sinned caused it than getting it fixed. Well, Jesus told his disciples, no one's sin caused the blindness. It was there for God's glory to become manifest in his life, apparent for all to see. Then Jesus healed that man. You see, there are some things that cannot be explained and trying to explain them becomes an exercise in futility. Sickness and disease were not a part of the original design. It came through sin however. So because of the imperfection that lives in the design through Adam's fall, illness can strike anyone with or without unrepented personal sin. God, being the wonderful and amazing God that He is, does not waste anything, even the bad things. Thus, in the kingdom of God, sickness and disease can either bring Him glory or bring us correction or both, but it is not wasted!

Chapter 11

WHAT HAS CONTROL?

Going back to an earlier point, if we are truly in the image of God, we too are three-fold beings. We are souls, energized and enlivened by a spirit and housed in bodies. If we don't understand our construction, we will often give control of our lives over to the pressure of illness. You see, while who we are is found in the essence of the soul, it is the spirit that is life. It must flow and commune with God. It is there that we receive strength, endurance, power. We live in a body. The body has its own tendencies and urges. It is carnal in nature. It is cursed by sin and is prone to illness, pain and suffering. Yet the spirit, that life-giving and restoration power, is from God. The soul, the essence of you, is free to decide which urges to follow, whether those of the spirit or those of the flesh, the carnal body. The question then becomes, what has control of us?

I dare not tell you that fighting illness is easy. For sure, it is probably one of the most difficult issues you'll face. It will challenge your faith on a continuous basis. But challenges make us stronger, quicker, wiser.

During a particularly low point in my life, namely during the time I suffered hallucinations, I began to feel like I might end up lost. There were times when the hallucinations were so mild that I could tell that I was hallucinating. But there were other times when the illusions were so strong that I could not distinguish the illusion from reality. I had conversations and interactions that still puzzle me to this very day. And in fact, after the hospitalization that detoxed my system of meds, I was terrified that I'd find out I'd said or done some really horrible things. Luckily that fear was unfounded but the fact that I was completely out of control of my own actions, thoughts and words still haunt me. It's like having your body invaded without your permission.

One issue with disease is that it tortures the weakest part of you. The flesh is the weakest part of mankind. It is the part that was given over to sin in Adam's fall. When your body is in pain and discomfort, there is a tendency to coddle that uncomfortable area. From the natural perspective, your primary focus becomes easing the dis-ease. You want to be pain-free, inflammation-free and back to normal as quickly and painlessly as possible. Sometimes though, that overwhelming desire is what gets in the way of our goal, which is freedom from disease.

The strongest enemy is the one that understands strength is relative. It takes more than sure force to win any war. When disease wages war against our bodies, often it comes in strong and overwhelming. But that is only the initial attack. Next it settles in and begins to wear you down. Pains, aches, swelling, discoloration and bruising, numbness, weakness, fatigue, nausea and a host of other symptoms work you over until you get tired and hopeless, depressed and desperate. It's a terrible process but that is the path of disease unless interrupted by faith and action, not to mention a lot of hope.

During the worst part of my disease, I was lucky enough to have tons of Facebook friends with similar illness and tons of faith and positive energy. That helped me regain control because constantly I was bombarded with messages of faith, dominion and hope. I had my family and friends pulling for me, reminding me of who I am. And so much came from it.

When we're sick, we have an illness. We are not that illness. We don't have to allow illness to change who we are. For so long, I was miserable. I felt sorry for myself. I thought the best part of my life was over because of all the limitations I had. All of a sudden I went from being an active, fit, young adult to being unable to walk through a grocery store without stopping repeatedly, wheezing, and feeling close to fainting. All of a sudden, my healthy 78 bpm heart rate was changed to 150 bpm and more at resting, extremely unhealthy. Everything changed and for a short season, I let that change me. Big mistake.

When you are challenged in your body and

that challenge remains unbeaten long enough, it can break your fighting spirit causing you to yield to disease and put your soul in distress. You lose control and it is then that sickness does the most damage.

Faith is often just a word to some, having yet to face something that caused them to depend solely upon the Lord. Often, we take credit for the work God has done. We credit good grades with being able to go to college. We credit college degrees with being able to find and keep a good job. We take credit for everything we can and expect others to celebrate us but we don't celebrate our Enabler... God is the enabler who gives you energy and strength and know-how in all situations and circumstances. It is by His very breath that we exist. Thus, to live as free and as victorious as He desired when He created us, we must have faith.

When I got sick, my faith became real to me, something that is as tangible in my heart as the blood that flows through it. And after I ran out of brute force ideas, I finally yielded first to the disease. Hopelessness flooded my very soul. But then somehow in all that despair, God gave me hope through others. And my faith came alive and today I am alive because of it, no doubt. By faith, I was able to turn over control to God. I had to ask myself some hard questions, whether I truly believed there is a "god" and what that would mean. I'd been preaching for a long time already, but preaching it and living it are different animals altogether. It all made sense to me when I stood to recite my knowledge of scripture. But at home, my emotions, desires and fears muddied the water. It skewed my vision and understanding of what I'd just taught to someone else. I had to face who I was and what I truly believed.

Fear has a tendency to scream at us, trying to overpower any courage that lives in our hearts. Then, almost in rhythm, it has a constant, nagging whisper of insecurities and previous failures. Fear hears the odds when you're diagnosed with a disease. It automatically tries to filter out any hope by constantly reminding you of who you are and what you "deserve" thus paralyzing your faith.

We must fight not to yield to our illnesses but we must also fight not to yield to our fears. It is when we feed our faith by denying our minds the leisure to ponder over the worst case scenarios that we begin to discover a hidden but life-changing power that dwells in us all. We become one of those rare individuals who live in natural bodies through supernatural faith and it is amazing once we walk fully into the place where God is in control.

Chapter 12
WHAT MUST DIE

No one's life fits neatly in a box and none of us are perfectly colored in without any of our essence flowing outside the line. We are complex creations, each with a specific purpose that is for sure going to be fulfilled with or without our help. Thus, this chapter isn't about specific issues of our hearts, but rather specifically about the general issues that hinder believers, particularly those who are health challenged already.

In my situation, the lengthiest process for me was discovering my unhealthy behaviors and thought processes. Often, we're so used to our negative, body-destroying behavior that we cannot pinpoint it on our own. We may know we yell too much, but we never bother to ask why we react with yelling, or tensing, or stress and pig out, or in my case, stress and nearly starve. We simply accept our reactions as a normal part of our lives and adjust. Our behavior then repeats itself over and over, becoming stronger in our minds each time and solidifying itself as a stronghold. Yes, that is how strongholds are created. And every stronghold must die. For those of us of the Faith, we understand that God is our Shelter, our Tower, our Banner and the One we run to when we are afraid. Anything else is like building an armory on sinking sand. It is only a matter of time.

For those who suffer with chronic and painful conditions such as lupus and fibromyalgia, you find yourself bed-ridden quite often with a lot of time to think. Often, we remember all the opportunities for a fuller life that was squandered. We remember our younger, healthier years and become saddened, hopeless and depressed. Each sad thought leads to deeper sadness until you find yourself buried without a ray of sunshine anywhere to be found. There, all sorts of darkness penetrate our hearts and minds. And for some, it gets so bad that they become oppressed. And oppression must die for us to walk in health, healing and wholeness.

An ill person has much more going on than some breakdown in the body or mind. In fact, we are so closely interwoven that nothing can affect one part of us without affecting the others. Some theologians and life specialists may disagree but indulge me for a brief time.

I can clearly remember times when I woke up in a great mood, ready to take charge of my day, but was then interrupted by pain or dysfunction in my body. That interruption bothered me enough that my mood shifted, my plans changed and adjustments were made. Even if I still went to work or continued on with my originally planned actions, the pain that was present with those actions certainly subtracted from the atmosphere of my day. To make it clearer, the Bible clearly teaches that sorrow of heart is rottenness to the bones.)

I'm not saying that all sad people are physically ill or that all physically ill people are sad and depressed. Quite to the contrary. But, for a physically ill person, they must battle the disease and the depression, the disease within a disease. It's easy to become sad when your body won't allow you to behave the way your spirit and mind wants you to. Depression can creep in when the body is instantly taken away from a mind that is still healthy and strong. So, people who are chronically ill will tell you that there is a constant war being fought to maintain peace of mind, hope and joy.

From the other perspective, people who are depressed, or who have various mental illnesses rarely can use their bodies to its full potential because their minds are not healthy. One sign of depression is decreased activity, not because of physical incapacity, but because of mental incapacity. You see, we're intimate creatures and each part needs the other part to operate efficiently.

Lastly, let's speak about the healthy spirit. When your spirit is healthy, it feeds life to your mind and body. But even with a healthy mind and body, if you are spiritually in darkness, you miss the best part of life. There are many of us who can testify to how empty we've felt even while we had everything, how lonely we felt even in a crowd of people. And all of that testifies to the power of a healthy spirit. Yes, to some degree you can think yourself better and feel a little better sometimes. Likewise, a sick body can drain the vigor from the mind. They are interwoven, neither much stronger than the other. But the spirit is stronger than both and has the power to transform both. And that is the essence of this book and particularly this chapter.

For the most part, people will agree that if you want something to grow, you must feed it. It has to be nurtured. It must be cared for, in other words. Plants grow with their food which is water and sunshine mixed with whatever nutrients are in the soil.

Now there are two important points that come to mind. The first is that we cannot feed ourselves anything. We need specific nutrients for specific issues and areas of our lives. The second is that faith and plants are a lot alike, which is why I used the above analogy. Most of us talk about faith, have heard of it, but have no clue how to use it or tap into it.

When you are fighting from a losing position, such as already being diagnosed with an illness, you have to work a little harder and sometimes wait just a little longer to see the results. I had to change how I behaved, how I thought, how I responded to life, what I ate and when I ate. I had to incorporate exercise and more sleep into my life. I had to begin to pay attention to myself and nurture myself. Illness forced me to begin loving myself, for which I'm grateful. No doubt, neglect was mostly responsible for my health issues.

Going backwards just a little, our faith isn't automatic. It's more like a muscle that must be used and developed. Like a plant, when our faith is in good soil, in God, it will grow and produce amazing things. It will carry us through life without fail. But when we misplace our faith and trust in worldly, temporal things, it fails us because people and things fail. We must feed our faith by reading the Bible and other spiritual books, associating with faith-filled people, and using it at every turn. Faith living must become a way of life.

When it comes to healing, it is as much a faith issue as it is a body issue. Now, I have to go on record to say that healing isn't about what issues doctors find in your body, not to me. It is about freedom from disease. These bodies are decaying and nothing can change that, no medicine in the world. Nevertheless, God is able to restore your health. He can remove all trace of disease and can alleviate any pain. Yet, not every person of faith with some chronic illness will be healed in this fashion. No preacher in the world can tell you the mind of God, why some are completely healed and others are only taught to allow God's grace to be sufficient. (See Paul's story)

What I can tell you is that the principles of God always work even if it does not manifest in the same way in every life. For me, some things were totally removed from me. Some things I had to learn to manage and control through faith and diligent care for myself. But either way, I know that the prayers being sent up for me were answered. I know that God healed me, particularly the parts that count.

My body is important. I must live in it for my entire life. But a broken body is just that. It can't keep me out of heaven. It won't send me to hell. It may impede my progress but as many heroic individuals have already shown, a broken body does not mean you cannot go on and live a full and happy life.

So while I awaited healing that I could feel, God was busy working with areas I paid little to no attention. He was dealing with my heart, my fears, my conceit, the lies that had penetrated my essence. Before I began to feel better, I actually became better. Pride died. After all, it's a bit difficult to have pride when you can't even bathe unsupervised. False humility died. When your spouse has to take complete care of you, you don't have to pretend to be humble anymore. When you hallucinate and lose control of what's going on in your life, you're as humbled as you can be. God pruned and purged until I thought I might die, but it wasn't until all the pruning was done that I began to see the healing that was promised in the Bible.

Chapter 13
THE ART OF WAR

When you begin to seek out something different than what you've ever had, you're going to face battles you've never before fought. But this is the art of war- no matter what battle you're fighting, the outcome remains the same if you are in faith and trusting God.

Soldiers are equipped for war. They're trained how to control their impulses. They're trained to watch, to report and to follow. They're given weapons and trained to use them. It doesn't stop when the fighting begins either. The training continues for new weapons, new strategies, etc. Things aren't much different in spiritual warfare either.

God teaches us through life experience, the testimony of others and through His Word. He equips us to stand and prevail in spiritual warfare. And make no mistake about it, sickness and disease creates warfare. Remember, God didn't originally design our bodies to break down. They were created to constantly renew themselves and hence last forever. It was sin that introduced sickness, disease and disabilities into human flesh. That knowledge is the first weapon in the arsenal of a believer.

As with anything, it is important to understand what is going on before responding. And sickness is not just a problem with the body and mind. It is a total system problem. And while your first priority may be to feel better, understand that this is warfare and it may get a little worse sometimes before it gets better. When you go to God for healing and relief, sometimes it may seem that He answered you with more pain and suffering. Maybe you've prayed and prayed about whatever illness you possess but it continued to get worse. But the worse mistake you can make right now is to prejudge the matter, or to lose hope. God is moving, just maybe not in the direction you hoped He would.

When I first began getting sick, I was in the throes of sin, committing adultery and was lost as to how to get free from all of the issues I had going on in my personal life. Rather quickly, Grave's disease swept into my life and derailed it. I hated that disease with a passion. It ruined everything in my mind. I was only days away from having IVF transfer to have children. That had to be postponed. I could no longer go grocery shopping, hang out for extended periods, or have sex without having severe chest pains, shortness of breath, extreme tiredness and more. I couldn't handle the heat. And because I was normally anemic, I couldn't handle the cold. I was simply miserable in my own body. It was like an invasion of the body snatchers moment. I was in there, but it did no good. I couldn't will myself better. I couldn't ignore it. And all the while, I had this lump growing in my neck, my eyes began to budge outward (as if they weren't already big enough), my skin roughened and my complexion darkened. So on top of being sick, I felt hideous.

The doctors told me I'd lose a lot of weight but instead I gained and plenty of it. I think at my heaviest, I was 192 pounds. My life had officially changed without my permission. And all I wanted was to restore some normalcy. But that was not the will of God for my healing. Being the stubborn person I am, I tried everything to take my life back. I didn't pay attention to my symptoms or what they could possibly mean. Even though I was a minister and knew the Bible like very few, I somehow was missing the voice of God in my illness telling me that it's time for me to heal, not my body which is going to decay one day anyway, but my soul. It was time for the me that is housed in this body to heal.

As I began to pay attention finally, I noticed that anger physically hurt me. I'd have bad chest pains and numbness when I was too upset. Worrying hurt me. I'd have bad headaches when I was stressing out. I could no longer walk around like I was Miss Thing either because I had a lump larger than an Adam's apple in my neck, impossible to hide. My skin looked terrible. I was always hot and sweating and uncomfortable and was gaining weight swiftly. Most times, I ended up bedridden. So all my days of conceit and vanity also ended. And as I began to pray and desperately beg God for healing, I began to realize that the parts of my life that ended because of my illness needed to end anyway. I had been warned to repent. I didn't and thus now, could it be that God was helping me by putting those limitations there that made me slow down and take note of who He is and who He had created me to be? I say absolutely!

It still took some years for me to get it, but looking back at the illnesses that attacked me and the changes they caused, I cannot say I regret ever becoming sick because sickness might have saved my soul. And for me, my soul is more important than my body. So when sickness was found in me, there came also warfare. I had a decision to make, fight God or fight with God. Accept it and learn from it, or keep fighting blindly without paying attention to what was going on and why. And that is the art of warfare- to understand the information put before you without trying to filter it through your emotions.

As you read this book, I'm sure you're looking for an answer to feel better right now, but that isn't the purpose of this book. This book is about being better for good rather than feeling better for a short season. You see, the battle you are facing is not going to be won by medications and doctors alone. It doesn't matter what illness it is (lupus, ms, grave's, cancer, heart disease, liver disease, kidney disease or something else), the outcome will depend much more upon you and the lifestyle changes you make rather than the pills you pop morning, noon and night.

Trust me, there was a time when I was on about 13-17 medications at one time. Some of those required that I take more than one pill at a time. Almost all of them were taken more than once a day. It was a mess and they didn't make me better at all. In fact, I could write another book on the dangers of medications. I had more medication interactions and bad reactions than I care to share. In fact, I had one pill that caused such severe hallucinations for me that twice I ended up in the hospital trying to figure out why with some person asking me if I "still" wanted to harm myself or others. It was terrifying! One pill caused severe amnesia. I was up, moving and doing, but remembered nothing, just brief foggy moments of recollection. Terrifying!

It was enough to convince me that there are many legal drugs that doctors prescribe that should be illegal. I've been intoxicated before and high on marijuana before, but they have medications that make a combo of alcohol and marijuana look like a walk in the park. I learned quickly that the medicines were not my saving grace or my pathway through the struggles in my body. I had to find another way.

My first big battle was pride and control. I didn't trust God as much as I thought I did. I tried all I could to change my situation through my own strength. But nothing made me better or changed the facts of my circumstances. I kept refusing the easiest answer, which is surrender, not to disease or dysfunction, but surrender to

God. Seems once you have totally surrendered to God, all other battles are made much easier because you are allowed to rest in Him while He guides your steps through the minefields of doubt, despair, pride, hopelessness and all other enemy emotions and responses that come to shake our faith in God. After all, the whole battle boils down to whether we love and trust our God no matter what it feels like to do so.

If you love, honor, obey and trust God, no illness in the world will ever prevail over you. Nothing will shake you because nothing can overcome your love born of faith in God. Make no mistake about it, love is the strongest force in this world and the one to come. And loving God is going to be the best thing you can do to overcome any challenge in this world. Though that sounds simple and perhaps even basic, it is the deepest revelation God has ever given me.

Now let's get into the meat of this book. Follow along with me through a brief journey that can help you learn to keep things in perspective, even while you're ill or in pain.

Chapter 14
Ooh, Tears of Pain

A tear can be born out of a physical need to cleanse the eyes or an emotional need to cleanse the soul. For the believer, there is a beautiful promise concerning our tears, that each one is bottled before our Lord.

The tears we shed are always for some purpose, and they are never wasted. From an emotional perspective, tears are essential for our well-being, but because there are so many negative ideas associated with tears, we spend most of our lives trying to avoid crying, trying to hide them away from the world. This is very unhealthy and leads to more problems emotionally. Suppression is not healing, nor is it conducive to it. It actually works against you, thus the worst thing to do is suppress your emotional upheavals. The better idea is to adapt coping mechanisms that allow for you to work through your issues without doing further damage to your psyche.

In the years of my most intense suffering, I'd hide myself away and cry a lot. I'd been falsely taught that tears were a sign of weakness and shouldn't be shared with anyone. I was taught to suppress my emotions. So indirectly, I was learning to lie to myself and fight against my own healing process, including the tears I had to shed.

Eventually, I came to the conclusion that it couldn't be wrong for me to cry. Since everyone does it, how could it be shameful? Bit by bit, I began to embrace myself, even the emotions that seemed to always be at odds. I embraced the pain I tried to run from. I embraced the shame, guilt and failures. It wasn't until I accepted that I will always be a perfectly imperfect vessel that I could focus on loving myself as I stood right then. Not for my potential. Not for who I was in the past. I had to love me in the moment. I had to be in the moment with myself to see what changes needed to be made in my life and to make them. I was an adult now and had to take responsibility first for myself.

When I was a child, I felt that tears should change things. I didn't understand why my parents weren't moved to act each time I cried. I thought crying would accomplish something in others. I didn't realize that those tears are for me, a cleansing of sorts that rids me of all the negative, painful, or selfish emotions that block me from hearing, seeing and accepting.

During some of my worst times, I would be in so much pain that I couldn't sit still but it hurt like the devil to move. I was dizzy on my feet, nauseated on my back. If I got too hot, I felt as if I was being suffocated. If I got too cold, my body ached as if every joint was arthritic. It got so bad that I felt totally uncomfortable in my own skin at all times. I rarely had a good moment. I ran back and forth to doctors and hospitals trying to figure out what was wrong. Each visit resulted in new prescriptions and different theories of why I was experiencing the pain. Soon, I lost hope that any doctor would actually listen to me. I think I cried every single day for over a month, shaking and aching, which also broke my spirit.

Some of you may be wondering why I didn't just bite the bullet and medicate myself more with painkillers. But I remember when pain pills were first introduced into the equation. Having come from a family where drug and alcohol abuse was prevalent, I was very reluctant to take the pills until absolutely necessary. I didn't want to turn into an addict. Turns out, my concerns were not unfounded. Over the course of six years, I was probably prescribed and given every major narcotic painkiller on the market and others. From hydrocodone to morphine to oxy, and then combo drugs like Fioricet with codeine, I was given a huge supply of all of it. In fact, I think it may have been slightly irresponsible of some hospitals to dole it out so freely, but in all fairness, it took the stronger stuff to control my pain many times.

Several times over the years, I found myself basically doped up and groggy and confused. It would come down to whether I wanted clarity but discomfort due to spasms and cramps and joint aches, or if I wanted some relief which would also mean being out of sorts as the meds worked themselves through my system. Each person with painful conditions has to make this same decision daily. Each of us has our own priorities. For me, it got to the point that relief provided through pain relievers was too high of a cost. I couldn't afford to be loopy and tired and drained. I couldn't afford the slight amnesic effects of some of the meds. I had to find another solution.

As I began to deal with pain on a natural level, I realized that every time we're in a great deal of pain, it feels like the worst pain ever. It's hard to remember something hurting more when you're in the throes of pain now. At least that was my experience. So each time I found myself folded up on my side whimpering, it felt as if I was reaching some new threshold of agony. In reality, I was not but I didn't realize it until I decided to go narcotics-free when treating my pain.

Pain is created when nerves react to inflammation or something else in the body. Basic over-the-counter painkillers have the same active anti-inflammatory ingredients that are also in narcotic pain meds most times. For instance, in hydrocodone pills, there is a certain amount of narcotics and a certain amount of acetaminophen, the same anti-inflammatory found in Tylenol and other over the counter meds. Thus, the narcotic effect is an added effect and while helpful at times, the primary issue is the inflammation that causes nerves to send pain signals to the brain. That can many times be handled with OTC meds. And in the case of Lupus, exercise is unbelievably helpful. There are foods with antioxidants and natural anti-inflammatory properties. While most of us do not want to do the legwork with figuring out what changes to make to our lifestyles, it is much better to handle pain naturally than to become dependent upon narcotic painkillers.

It wasn't a quick or easy journey, and it was riddled with tears, but I am glad to be able to write this book and share my story with clarity.

Pain pills, depression meds and anti-anxiety pills do not have to be your destiny.

Chapter 15

The Second Tear

The struggle of daily life with an incurable disease is different each moment, completely unpredictable at times. When that disease causes pain levels above an ache throughout the day, the struggle multiplies.

I remember the beginning when my fingers would cramp, ache and then freeze up in pain. I was terrified I had carpal tunnel or some horrible condition like rheumatoid arthritis. My typing speed slowed. I struggled more and more with daily function. Sweeping, mopping, washing dishes and even driving became painful when my joints were inflamed. Sometimes, the painkillers would help and sometimes they wouldn't.

It didn't take me long to figure out that my life was going to change. I didn't have a choice about it. That hurt more than anything. I had to change my life and adjust my goals. I had to... had to... had to. It felt like prison and that is the point of this chapter. Illness and prison both represent the same thing, lack of freedom. Both bring about a certain amount of physical bondage and that's an ordeal all by itself.

As a person who has been told what I can no longer eat, drink or what activities I probably need to avoid, I understand how it feels for a person to limit you when your mind and heart does not feel limited. It's so easy to slip into despising your body for holding you back. But those negative emotions and attitudes are often part of the problem and makes things worse rather than better. It's difficult to love yourself when you feel like you're imprisoned in a body you don't want or that you feel has failed you. But that perspective will keep you sick, depressed and powerless. Staying positive is important, and the more painful the condition, the more important it becomes. Joy is a conduit to healing, health and wholeness.

I remember one day I'd been in bed all day. Pain was screaming through my body. I'd been crying off and on all day. Yet, when my family arrived, their jokes and stories of their day made me laugh. And even though the pain didn't go away, my spirits lifted and suddenly it didn't seem so unbearable. The medicine of a happy heart cannot be overstated. And frankly, it is the only weapon we have against the suffocation of tears.

Chapter 16
The Wash

There aren't a lot of resources to teach you how to deal with humiliation. The fact is, shame can be one of the biggest hindrances to rebuilding a beautiful life. Sometimes because of what has happened to us, what we've done and what we failed to do can plague us in the back of our minds, making us question our value as human beings.

During the beginning of my walk with God, I used to feel so ragged by the heart when I read the Bible. Every page convicted me of crimes and I felt condemned, low and unworthy. Is there any wonder that the Bible itself says the Word kills but the Spirit gives life. I couldn't handle all the guilt. I wanted the freedom, light yoke and peace promised in the Bible. I wanted to walk in my call, close to God and free from sin. Unfortunately, each time I had opportunity, I found a reason that I didn't deserve any of it. So because of the humiliation of my past, I kept sabotaging the plan of God in my life and forfeiting the promises. I couldn't receive because I had not yet been cleansed of my guilt conscience. I hadn't allowed it.

The process of forgiveness must necessarily include the washing of the conscience, a repair if you will, to the psyche of the person who God has forgiven, teaching them to extend that same forgiveness unconditionally, the same way it was originally given to us. Without restraint, God promises us eternal redemption. Without condition, He pours his love and mercy upon us. And in that same way, he want us to be agents of his love and mercy to others. But to do that, we must be totally free. We cannot be bound in our hearts and minds to the old person, old life, or old decisions.

When you have done some things you're not proud of, even when others don't know about it, there is a tendency to be fearful of what others think and know. But the truth is, the root issue is what you think and know. Sometimes, we believe others are judging us when in reality, the condemnation is coming from within. Indeed, no one can make you feel condemned but you. And usually, it comes from some deep seated guilt in your heart.

No one on this planet is without guilt because no one on this planet is perfect. We all make mistakes. We all do things we shouldn't do, and have done things wrong on purpose. Sometimes, the enemy of our souls try to take advantage of that guilty conscience that hadn't been washed by the pure blood of Jesus Christ and makes us feel unworthy. He plants thoughts that make us feel so low that not even the love of God and all His mercy can touch or cure. But it is all a lie. There is nothing that the love of God cannot heal. No past mistake so horrible that God cannot forgive it. And if God does not condemn you, then why continue on condemning yourself, walking in humiliation?

When we have all that bad stuff bound up in our hearts, the body shows it eventually in a host of major and minor illnesses. I mean, if you look at the majority of known illnesses today, they are caused by or worsened by stress. Guilt, humiliation, shame causes stress. We have to let it go and be healed in the mind and spirit, and then the body. If science has proven anything, it has proven the power of spirituality in healing. It has proven the need for emotional stability in healing. It has proven that we are so delicately interwoven that any issue in one area affects them all over time. It has taught us to identify and deal with our problems, even the emotional ones.

Chapter 17

EMOTIONS ARE NOT THE ENEMY

It may seem that all those feelings are the problem. It may seem that without all the emotional upheavals, life would be better. But here is a case for emotions.

I personally don't believe there is any flaw in the human design. Even those sometimes pesky emotions have a purpose. They create balance and attachment. The depth of human emotions can defy explanation. Somehow, we can experience a myriad of conflicting emotions simultaneously. We can be happy but grief-stricken, all while being proud but feeling humbled. We often vacillate between conflicting emotions, trying to find some sort of balance. We wrestle with our emotions as if they are the enemy. They are not the enemy.

Emotion is an indicator of your position in life. It points out the adjustments that are and are not working. If you are participating in activity that causes emotional upheaval, that is your inner truth trying to call attention to the actions, thoughts or words. Your inner truth is your life force, programmed with destiny and purpose. When our actions, atmosphere and thoughts begin to stray away from that, it creates conflict in the soul (mind, will, emotions). So when we start to feel a "certain kind of way" about life, people, ourselves, the feeling is not the enemy. It is simply an indicator that something is off and preventing a positive exchange between our soul, spirit and body. Interruptions of energy flow causes problems, even health problems. It is just that serious. It is also just that simple. Our responsibility is to be true to ourselves, our creation purposes. When we get off in some way, our alarm system goes crazy. Our emotions fall out of whack. Our thoughts become unstable and our actions show the imbalance in our lives.

Illness is simply miscommunication in the

body. The body is designed to keep out harmful substances and to pass off toxins so that we're able to use the good in the things we ingest and pass off the bad. When the body is not properly communicating, it will allow in things that shouldn't be. It will not attack what should be attacked, or sometimes it will read as harmful an organ or something necessary to the body and attack it. For instance, autoimmune disorders are when your body misreads signals from your internal organs and attack them as foreign. Immunodeficiency disorders are when the body cannot protect itself because the proper signals that alert the brain to issues in the body are not firing.

Chapter 18
The Love Shift

I still remember the night that I realized how much hatred and anger I held for myself, how ashamed I was inside. I remember looking at myself in the mirror and feeling despair. But in the middle of all those tears, I realized that for all the grieving I was going through, I was still alive. As much as it felt like the pain would swallow me whole, I was still here. I was not actually suffocating. I was still breathing quite fine.

So, at that point, I realized that the paralysis that comes from pain is an illusion. The stagnation we experience, the dramatic effects in the brain, is all an emotional illusion that draws me in and keeps me from actually operating effectively in the real world. And that illusion had to end.

I stood there with tears streaming, cascading down my face, neck and covering my chest. I could barely see. Still, I grabbed a towel and wet it and began washing my face. I squared my shoulders and looked myself in the eyes. The kindest thing I could manage and mean at the time was, "I will love you if no one else does." And that was the beginning of a better life for me.

It didn't happen overnight, but I learned to be emotionally honest with myself and I embraced true friends who would hold me accountable to do so. I faced the destructive behavior I'd practiced so long. I faced the judgments I'd embraced about the mistakes I'd made in life. I faced the pain of falling short of my own potential. And I submitted those thoughts and opinions and mistakes and missteps to the Lord for safe keeping, for Him to work in it all so that my life could be complete, so that I could be free.

There was one particular point in my life that I literally felt like I was coming apart at the seams. I had so much held inside that I could no longer compartmentalize. Everything hurt. Everything bothered me. Everything triggered me. I couldn't discern where the root was because I'd allowed the infection to become systematic. I was emotionally out of whack. I was physically out of whack. There was no agreement in my temple. And so, it began to fall apart.

When you're emotionally confused and overwhelmed, it is quite difficult to find your way out. The only thing that can point you through it is honest surrender and acceptance. Seems when we wrestle to keep it together, to appear normal, to resist the changes that are happening in us, that is when we hurt the most and the most damage is inflicted to our psyche which plays out in our bodies. But when we decide to own our brokenness and pain, we are then empowered to deal with it.

I know you've heard a thousand different things concerning your emotions. You've read the books. You've listened to the experts and those who profess to live a balanced life. But seems you cannot find a system that works for you. That's because no one can tell you a detailed plan to deal with your emotions since no one could ever truly understand all the factors that play a part of your emotional makeup. Even those who have endured similar situations did not perceive it the same as you did, thus there will always be fundamental differences and what worked like a charm for them will need a tremendous amount of tweaking to work for you. Thus, I don't teach plans. I teach principles. I teach the fundamentals of healing, applicable to anyone. It is my desire to share the principles that can be applied and reapplied as needed.

Concerning your emotions, fighting them is not the answer. Embracing them is how you deal with them. Remember, you are the captain of this ship. Your emotions are your choice, even if made within a fraction of a second. You don't control your emotions. You train them. You bring them into agreement with your core values. Emotions, after all, are an asset to who you are, not the sum total of who you are.

Chapter 19
The ME Decision

When I decided to heal, it wasn't about techniques and programs. It wasn't about religion. It wasn't about anyone else. It was about me. It was about me making a decision to truly give it a try, my faith that is. After ten years, I was weary trying to act the part of "saved" and trying to meet the expectations of my Christian peers. I was worn out with all the personal battles and public failures and the general state of defeat I was living in. No doubt, my body deciding to breakdown was very significant for me because it was only outwardly mimicking the dysfunction that was going on inside.

So the day finally came when I decided either this faith was real or false. I was tired of trying to convince the world when I wasn't totally convinced that God's way was the right way as outlined in the Bible. And trust me, the Bible is but an outline. You're going to live the meat of it all. The story is yours to write in honor of God and His Christ who righted our wrongs.

According to my faith, the same path that provided salvation and redemption also provided healing and peace. Why should I believe the rather intangible ones like salvation and redemption if I couldn't believe the more tangible and proveable ones like healing and peace? So, I put it all down, the whole religious system of peer control that I'd learned. I put down my facade. No masks. No lies. No more denial. I admitted my brokenness. I admitted that I still had no clue and that the principles I was teaching others was not working for me. I wasn't sure if the failure was in my application or in my understanding of the principles. I even opened myself again to the idea that maybe the issue was with the principles themselves, that I'd embraced a lie.

I was open to anything. That may sound

bad, but it took all that for me to get healed. I had to go back to the basics and restore myself from the core of my being, which meant asking the hard questions and facing them. I knew for sure that sickness at a young age was not going to work for me. I was not willing to accept it no matter what it cost me to heal.

Somehow in most things in life, if you feel that something must work, it usually does. Why? Because you mentally remove the option of failure, because you decide not to accept sameness or worsened conditions as the final answer. Thus, you work your plan, adjust it and rework it until you get improved results. That's what I had to do spiritually to find the wisdom nuggets I share in this book.

One of the first realizations that came was how religious I truly was. I had a Bible scripture for everything but very few real testimonies of how well they worked. I was overly religious, hiding behind church rather than being in Christ. He'd become nothing more than a shield for my brokenness. He was empty rhetoric in my mouth. I'd adopted a form of godliness but was denying the power thereof. I had the dresses, the speech and the routine down to a science. But there was no real power in my life. There were only minute amounts of change. There was no promised joy or peace. There was no freedom. In fact, I felt more in bondage because of my faith. Then with the illnesses, I utterly felt rejected. But thankfully, we do not and cannot walk on feelings alone.

As my body continued on a downward spiral, I soon realized that my only hope did not lie in pharmaceuticals. There was no true hope in traditional medicine. They were telling me that Lupus is a lifelong battle. Grave's disease can be a lifelong battle causing me to be medicated the rest of my life, first to destroy the thyroid and then to replace the thyroid hormone. Epilepsy was also said to be permanent. I knew that I didn't want to spend the rest of my youth or life in and out of hospitals. So I turned to my faith once more. If there was any hope of restoration, I knew it had to be through faith. It was my last resort, my last hope, so it had to work.

I began reading my Bible once again. I still

believed that one book had more to it than I'd gotten from the first few reads. Somehow, being at such a hard point opened me up to all possibilities, including the one that I'd not chosen the right faith.

I began at the beginning, analyzing the words I read as if I'd never heard them before. And as I read, a whole new faith opened to me. It was one without all those restrictions. It was a faith of freedom and supply, abundance even in times of suffering. It was a faith of love and compassion, mercy and acceptance, renewal and redemption. All the chains that were on my heart and mind began to fall away. The boundaries I'd previously embraced that limited me from walking in the fullness of God's power was now gone. And all in one scripture, I was set free mentally and my healing began with the scripture that informs us that with God all things are possible.

With God, all things are possible is not a guarantee, as I once figured my healing should be. I thought I should be automatically healed as soon as I present an illness before God, but the

Bible doesn't support that common misconception of healing. So there I was having the Bible disprove my previous understanding of it as taught to me by various teachers I'd had. It was no fault of theirs that the Word was not previously working in my life. After all, faith is very personal and we have the responsibility to find information and truth. We cannot be so lazy as to expect any one teacher to be able to relieve us of the duty of personal study and devotion with God.

I realize that everything that is coming after this sentence is going to sound foreign to you, but bare with me for the remainder of the this book. Read with an open mind and heart.

Sickness and disease, as we previously discussed, happens when either a foreign object invades the body or when there is a miscommunication in the body. Often, miscommunications happen as various body parts begin to wear out due to misuse or malnourishment. Thus, to fix sickness and disease, harmful foreign objects must be removed and balance must be restored to the body. It must be nourished on every level from emotional to natural. Any breakdown will force undue stress on the rest of the body because we are fully integrated beings.

Each system depends upon the other to create a cycle of renewal and wellness. Our bodies were not originally created to fail or die. Originally, we were designed for eternal life, meaning the design itself was flawless. Our system of intake and output is perfect for ridding our bodies of unnecessary substances. Our nervous systems are the fastest relay systems known to man, with our brains processing a dizzying amount of information per millisecond. In short, your body is the most sophisticated computer system in the world.

Nothing in existence is more delicate than the body, than the creation of man. Still, most of our design is a mystery even to us. But everything you need to heal and be restored is already in you and it has to begin with that central nervous system, the core of your being, your brain. For spiritual purposes, let's say your mind. In your mind, balance has to be restored.

There's a well known, but mostly unspoken fact in the community of the chronically or terminally ill. Seems you're only mildly ill until you find out what you have. Then, symptoms you never noticed before or that actually were not there before, come from out of nowhere. All of a sudden, the mild stomach upset that caused you indigestion now causes severe pain because you know you have ulcers. You know how painful they are, how dangerous they can be. So no sooner than the diagnosis comes, you find yourself feeling worse, even when you try to block it mentally with denial or feel good thoughts.

Why does cancer seem more dire after the diagnosis than before? Because you mind plays a tremendous role in what goes on in your body. There are documented cases of people with psychosomatic illnesses, even psychosomatic pregnancies that went all the way up until the point of an empty labor. The mind is just that powerful. Left uncontrolled and undirected, the mind can be your biggest enemy to your healing.

But when the mind is brought under control, you can direct that focus toward creating a balanced state. A balanced state is where healing happens and wholeness dwells.

The thought of all the years of bondage I lived before I joined church and all the bondage afterwards trying to be an acceptable believer brings tears to my eyes. It is unfortunate that so many of us who came to God with an open heart and a desperate love find ourselves disillusioned by the disappointment inherent in religion. I was there. But it wasn't until sickness that I was forced to address everything in my life, not just the sickness in the body but the sickness in the mind and spirit as well. It breaks my heart that so many of us are diseased in our bodies, minds and spirits. But I'm encouraged that I've been there and am a testimony of what true relationship with God can do. So writing this book is my way of being proactive for those who suffer, my way of showing gratitude for what GOD did through faith.

Chapter 20
That Think Link

You know this next statement to be true, but you hadn't spent enough time meditating upon it. Your brain is your body's control center. When there is an issue in the body, the brain is also affected. Thus when there is a problem in the body, part of healing has to happen in the mind, in the thinking and imagination. How we think directly affects our bodies.

MIND, WILL, EMOTIONS= SOUL

During one point of my illness, I was going through so much physically that I'd given up hope. I think I was just waiting to die. Didn't seem the pain would ever abate. Didn't seem medication could help. Didn't seem there was hope in anything, including prayer. But after awhile, I began to pray a different prayer. Instead of begging God to take the disease out of my body, I began to thank Him for the fact that in spite of all the bad diagnoses and the pain in my body and the medication interactions, I was still alive, still mentally functioning and had people who loved me enough to believe for me while I felt too weak to believe for myself.

After I stopped begging and denying my plight, once I accepted that I was sick physically and broken emotionally, THEN something happened. At the point of surrender, my perspective began changing. I'd spent too much of my life energy focusing on things I couldn't control, trying to get things I didn't need, or hold on to people who were not meant to stay.

For all the striving in my life, it was at the point of surrender that I realized how meaningless it all was. I mean really, how useful was a lot of money if you're too sick to enjoy it? How sorrowful to have tons of friends sit around and helplessly watch you suffer and then die? It was meaningless, everything that I'd jeopardized my health for, because even though I'd gotten to my goal, I'd given away something just as precious. It was in surrender that I found the truth, that I had dishonored myself while seeking to please and serve others. I thought it was too late for me, but then everything began to change. There isn't a day that goes by that I'm not grateful for the spiritual shift that led to wholeness in my life. And that shift began in mind.

You must understand, how we process information controls every aspect of our lives. Stinking thinking stinks up your entire life. For some of you, when you're hurting, you feel like crap so you begin to think crappy thoughts which lead to crappy words that create more crap in your life. So, if that is the creative cycle, the adjustment has to come to the mind.

There are many healers and doctors writing books and finally acknowledging the mind's role in physical healing. Some recommend meditation and chanting. Personally, I use affirmations and meditation. They brought amazing change into my mind, heart, words and life.

It's extremely difficult to feel blue when you are using words to guide your thoughts and infiltrating your heart with what you desire, and with good, clean and empowering words. Remember, words are creative power, spoken from the heart. The heart is filled with what you see and what you hear (words). Even faith comes by hearing (words). So words are both the beginning and the end. Everything in between is the think link.

It's important to speak the right things, and to think on them. Read the right things, and think on them. Meditate upon what you hope for, and speak about it. Eventually, this positive cycle squeezes out all disagreement from your life: people, places, and actual illnesses.

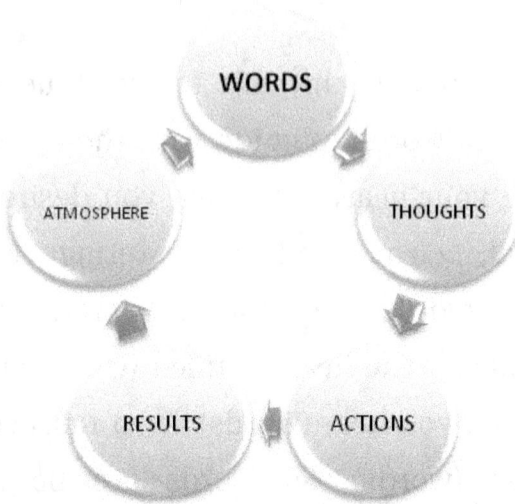

When you begin to understand this cycle, you put yourself in a position to change everything, not just your physical situation, but anything else you don't particularly care for. The easiest place to begin to interrupt negative cycles is words.

When you first start saying the right things, it won't be because you see them. But if you continue to speak them, they will enter your life cycle and begin changing everything.

Epilogue
RESTORATION

Healing is not a straight path. There are a lot of steps forward and a few setbacks, but if you stick with truth with a determination to set right any area that isn't, you will reach wholeness. Not always when you reach that place does your medical records reflect it, but you'll know it beyond a shadow of a doubt.

I was sick for so long that I cannot pinpoint the day my body began to heal itself, or the first day without symptoms. By the time the healing began, I was so wrapped up in correcting the thoughts that led there that I'd lost touch with much of the issues in my body anyway. It just seems like I woke up okay one day and have been okay since. Sure, I have days when the symptoms come but the chains of sickness do not shackle me anymore.

Restoration is an experience that requires courage and honesty. You must be courageous enough to face the truth about any brokenness in your life. Think of it this way: if you cannot be honest with yourself, who can you be honest with?

Restoration denotes a re-establishment of something, a reinstatement or return of some kind. As it pertains to health, restoration is a return to wholeness. As it pertains to your emotions, it is a reinstatement of your dominion, your ability to choose how you will feel, and thus what you will do. Remember, these bodies and this life are all about cohesion. If you aren't restored on every level, then you hadn't truly been restored. It's important that you don't leave any of yourself behind on your journey to wholeness, health and happiness. You are not a fragmented creature. You are a multi-faceted creature with endless potential for growth, recreation and fullness. When you see yourself as one unit, love yourself fully as one unit, then you are for sure free from any bondage at all, no matter what you've been through physically or emotionally. That's the purpose of this book, to make sure you are free from the bondage of a broken body, damaged emotions and spiritual malnourishment.

You may need to read this book several times, as well as find other holistic approach information to help you retrain your thinking, words and behavior with yourself. Fact of the matter is, if loving self were easy all the time, no one would need to write a book, and most pharmacies would be out of a job. I am convinced that self-love put into practice is powerful enough to shift everything, even something as debilitating as cancer, lupus or epilepsy. I'm walking in it day by day, and I hope to hear your stories of healing. I know it works. Will you let the cascade of tears flowing from you wash you of every impurity that defiles your body, emotions and spirit? I certainly hope so. It is the ultimate act of self-love.

Other Books by the Author

-*The Rape of Innocence: Taking Captivity Captive*

-*Becoming: My Personal Memoirs*

-*Tangled*

-*Poetic Infinity: Passion and Promise*

-*Raw Redemption*

-*Unnecessary Roughness*

-*A Heart in Motion*

-*Heart Strings*

-*The Path to Oneness*

-*The Ultimate Survival Guide for the Entrepreneurial Woman*

-*Black Dakota*

-*The Snare of a Strange Woman*

-*Truth and Intimacy: A Couple's Journal*

-*In the Presence of Pain*

-*Meet, Greet, and Get Rich*

-*The Network Marketing Millionaire*

Lanico Media House Books

-*Nine Angels by Tom Henry*
-*The Adventures of Delilah Daisy: Delilah's Big Adventure by Cegi Farmer*
-*Forgetting My First Love by Derrick S. Farris*
-*My Life in Devotion by Angela Dockter*
-*Inner Sanctum by Darlene Oakley*
-*The Asquinn Twins: No Greener Pastures by Heather Radford*

www.ingramcontent.com/pod-product-compliance
Lightning Source LLC
Chambersburg PA
CBHW062100270326
41931CB00013B/3157